AGEING WELL AND STAYING HEALTHY:

Healthy ageing

Victoria T. Patton

Copyright

TABLE OF CONTENTS

Introduction

While wellbeing is regularly found to be higher in later life than among young or middle-aged persons, it is subsequently found to fall in the oldest elderly, despite the fact that advancing age is linked with physical and cognitive impairment.

Future subjective health is predicted by affective, eudemonic, and evaluative wellbeing, indicating that decreased wellbeing is not only a byproduct of ill health but is also systematically linked to the emergence of poor health.

Social interactions have a greater impact on mortality than physical inactivity and obesity, and are equivalent to other known mortality risk factors like smoking and alcohol usage.

Greater happiness of life was linked to survival for an average of more than nine years. Effects were significant, withThe risk of death is around three times higher for those who enjoy life to the lowest (as opposed to maximum) third.

CHAPTER ONE

HOW TO STAY OLD AND STAY HEALTHY.

Numerous factors impact healthy aging. Some of these, similar as genetics, aren't in our control. Others - like exercise, a healthy diet, going to the croaker regularly, and taking care of our internal health - are within our reach.

v Get moving Exercise and physical exertion
v Healthy eating Make smart food choices
v Getting a good night's sleep
v Quit smoking
v Alcohol and other substances
v Go to the croaker
v Social insulation and loneliness
v Stress
v Depression and overall mood
v Rest conditioning and pursuits
v How different factors affect cognitive health
v How cognitive training affects health issues
v Taking care of your physical health

While scientists continue to laboriously probe how to decelerate or help age-affiliated declines in physical health, they've formerly discovered multiple ways to ameliorate the chances of maintaining optimal health latterly in life. Taking care of your physical health involves staying active, making healthy food choices, getting enough sleep, limiting your alcohol input, and proactively managing your health care. Little changes in each of these areas can go a long way to support healthy aging.

Get moving Exercise and physical exertion
Whether you love it or detest it, physical exertion is a foundation of healthy aging. Scientific substantiation suggests that people who exercise regularly not only live longer but also may live more — meaning they enjoy further times of life without pain or disability. Aged grown-up, in a demesne, doing yoga on a mat

A study of grown-ups 40 and aged set up that taking 8,000 way or further per day, compared to only taking 4,000 way, was associated with a 51 lower threat of death from all causes. You can increase the number of way you get each day by doing conditioning that keep your body moving, similar as gardening, walking the canine, and taking the stairs rather of the elevator.

Although it has numerous other benefits, exercise is an essential tool for maintaining a healthy weight. Grown-ups with rotundity have an increased threat of death, disability, and numerous conditions similar as type 2 diabetes and high blood pressure. Still, thinner isn't always healthier moreover. Being or getting too thin as an aged grown-up can weaken your vulnerable system, increase the threat of bone fracture, and in some cases may be a symptom of the complaint. Both rotundity and light conditions can lead to loss of muscle mass, which may beget a person to feel weak and fluently worn out.

As people age, muscle function frequently declines. Aged grown-ups may not have the energy to do everyday conditioning and can lose their independence. Still, exercise can help aged grown-ups maintain muscle mass as they progress. In a 2019 disquisition of data from NIA's Baltimore Longitudinal Study of Aging, experimenters set up that moderate to vigorous physical exertion is explosively associated with muscle function, anyhow of age. This suggests that exercise may be suitable to help age- related decline in muscle function.

In addition to helping aged grown-ups live more, maintaining muscle mass can help them live longer. In another study, experimenters set up that in grown-ups aged than 55, muscle mass was a better predictor of life than weight or body mass indicator (BMI).
Although numerous studies concentrate on the goods of physical exertion on weight and BMI, exploration has set up that indeed if you're not losing weight, exercise can still help you live longer and more. There are numerous ways to get started. Try being physically active in short spurts always or setting aside specific times each week to exercise. Numerous conditioning, similar as brisk walking or yoga, are free or low-cost and don't bear special outfit. As you come more active, you'll start feeling reenergized and refreshed after exercising rather of exhausted. The key is to find ways to get motivated and keep going.

Healthy eating Make smart food choices

Making smart food choices can help cover you from certain health problems as you age and may indeed help ameliorate brain function. As with exercise, eating well isn't just about your weight. With so numerous many different diets out there, choosing what to eat can be confusing. The 2020- 2025 Dietary Guidelines for Americans give healthy eating recommendations for each stage of life. The Dietary Guidelines suggest an eating ways with lots of fresh fruits and vegetables, whole grains, healthy fats, and spare proteins. Regale plate on a table with salmon and veggies important of the exploration shows that the Mediterranean- style eating pattern, which includes fresh yield, whole grains, and healthy fats, but lower dairy and further fish than a traditional American diet, may have an impact on health. A 2021 study assaying the eating patterns of further than 21,000 actors set up that people nearly following the Mediterranean- style pattern had a significantly lower threat of unforeseen cardiac death.

A low- swab diet called Dietary Approaches to Stop Hypertension (gusto) has also been shown to deliver significant health benefits. Studies testing the DASH diet set up that it lowers blood pressure, helps people lose weight, and reduces the threat of type 2 diabetes and heart complaint.

Yet another eating pattern that may support healthy aging is the MIND diet, which combines a Mediterranean- style eating pattern with gusto. Experimenters have set up that people who nearly follow the MIND diet have better overall cognition — the capability to suppose, learn, and flash back — compared to those with other eating styles.

Try starting with small changes by espousing one or two aspects of the Mediterranean- style eating pattern or MIND diet. Several studies have shown that incorporating indeed a part of these eating patterns, similar as further fish or further lush flora, into your diurnal eating habits can ameliorate health issues. One study of 182 aged grown-ups with frequent migraines set up that a diet lower in vegetable oil painting and advanced in adipose fish could reduce migraine headaches. Another study that followed nearly 1,000 aged grown-ups over five times set up that consumption of green lush vegetables was significantly associated with slower cognitive decline.

Getting a good night's sleep

Getting enough sleep helps you stay healthy and alert. Indeed though aged grown-ups need the same seven to nine hours of sleep as all grown-ups, they frequently do not get enough. Feeling sick or being in pain can make it harder to sleep, and some drugs can keep you awake. Not getting enough quality sleep can make a person perverse, depressed, absentminded, and more likely to have cascade or other accidents. Aged grown-ups sleeping in a bed
 Sleep quality matters for memory and mood. In one study of grown-ups aged than 65, experimenters set up that those who had poor sleep quality had a harder time problem- working and concentrating than those who got good quality sleep. Another study, which looked at data from nearly 8,000 people, showed that those in their 50s and 60s who got six hours of sleep. This may be because shy sleep is associated with the buildup of beta- amyloid, a protein involved in Alzheimer's complaint. Poor sleep may also worsen depression symptoms in aged grown-ups. Arising substantiation suggests that aged grown-ups who were diagnosed with depression in the history, and don't get quality sleep, may be more likely to witness their depression symptoms again.

 More generally, a 2021 study set up that aged grown-ups who didn't sleep well and napped frequently were at lesser threat of dying within the coming five times. Again, getting good sleep is associated with lower rates of insulin resistance, heart complaint, and rotundity. Sleep can also ameliorate your creativity and decision- making chops, and indeed your blood sugar situations.

 What can you do?
There are numerous affects you can do to help you sleep better, similar as following a regular sleep schedule. Try to fall

asleep and get up at the same time every day. Avoid napping late in the day, as this may keep you awake at night. Exercise can help you sleep better, too, if it is n't too close to bedtime. Research suggests that behavioral interventions, similar as awareness contemplation, can also ameliorate sleep quality.

Quit smoking

It does n't count how old you're or how long you 've been smoking, exploration confirms that indeed if you 're 60 or aged and have been smoking for decades, quitting will ameliorate your health. Quitting smoking at any age will lower your threat of cancer, heart attack, stroke, and lung complaint.
 Ameliorate your blood rotation
 Ameliorate your sense of taste and smell
 Increase your capability to exercise
 Set a healthy illustration for others
One study set up that among men 55 to 74 times old and women 60 to 74 times old, current smokers were three times more likely to die within the six- time follow-up period than those who had noway smoked.

Still, quit, if you bomb. Quitting smoking is good for your health and may add times to your life. One study of nearly 200,000 people demonstrated that aged grown-ups who quit smoking between the periods of 45 and 54 lived about six times longer compared to those who continued to bomb. Grown-ups who quit between the periods of 55 to 64 lived about four times longer. It's noway too late to stop smoking and reap the benefits of breathing easier, having further energy, saving plutocrat, and perfecting your health.

Alcohol and other substances

Like all grown-ups, aged grown-ups should avoid or limit alcohol consumption. Aging can lead to social and physical changes that make aged grown-ups more susceptible to alcohol abuse and abuse and more vulnerable to the consequences of alcohol. heavy drinking affects every organ in the body, including the brain.
A comprehensive study from the National Institute on Alcohol Abuse and Drunkenness shows that alcohol consumption among aged grown-ups, especially women, is on the rise. The experimenters also set up substantiation that certain brain regions show signs of unseasonable aging in alcohol-dependent men and women. In addition, heavy drinking for extended ages in aged grown-ups may contribute to poor heart health, as shown in this 2016 study. These studies suggest that stopping or limiting the use of alcohol could ameliorate heart health and help the accelerated aging seen with heavy alcohol use.
In addition to being conservative with alcohol, aged grown-ups and their caregivers should be apprehensive of other substances that can be misused or abused. Because aged grown-ups are generally specified opioids for pain and benzodiazepines for anxiety or trouble sleeping, they may be at threat for abuse and dependence on these substances. One study of grown-ups progressed 50 and aged showed that abuse of tradition opioids or benzodiazepines is associated with studies of self-murder.
If you or a loved one needs help with substance abuse or alcohol use. You can also try chancing a support group for aged grown-ups with substance or alcohol abuse issues.

Go to the croaker

Going to the croaker for regular health wireworks is essential for healthy aging. A 2021 study set up that getting regular check- ups helps croakers catch habitual conditions beforehand and can help cases reduce threat factors for complaint, similar as high blood pressure and cholesterol situations. People who went to the croaker regularly also reported advanced quality of life and passions of heartiness. Aged adult reviewing information with his croaker
In recent times, scientists have developed and bettered upon laboratory, imaging, and analogous natural tests that help uncover and cover signs of age- related complaint. Dangerous changes in the cells and motes of your body may do times before you start to witness any symptoms of the complaint. Tests that descry these changes can help medical professionals diagnose and treat a complaint beforehand, perfecting health issues. At least monthly and conceivably more depending on your health. You cannot reap the benefits of medical advancements without regular passages to the croaker for physical examinations and other tests. Regular wireworks can uncover conditions and conditions you may not yet be apprehensive of, similar as diabetes, cancer, and cardiovascular disease. However, you may lose the chance of having your croaker
 catch a complaint in its foremost stages, when it would be most treatable, If you only seek medical attention when you 're passing symptoms. Regular check- ups can help insure you could start treatment months or times before than would have been possible else.

Taking care of your internal health

Mental health, or internal heartiness, is essential to your overall health and quality of life. It affects how we suppose, feel, act, make choices, and relate to others. Managing social insulation, loneliness, stress, depression, and mood through medical and tone- care is crucial to healthy aging.

Social insulation and loneliness

As people age, changes similar as hail and vision loss, memory loss, disability, trouble getting around, and the loss of family and musketeers can make it delicate to maintain social connections. This makes aged grown-ups more likely to be socially insulated or to feel lonely. Although they sound analogous, social insulation and loneliness are different. Loneliness is the distressing feeling of being alone or promised, while social insulation is the lack of social connections and having many people to interact with regularly. An aged woman, appearing sad, looking out a window

Several recent studies show that aged grown-ups who are socially insulated or feel lonely are at advanced threat for heart complaint, depression, and cognitive decline. A 2021 study of further than 11,000 grown-ups aged than age 70 set up that loneliness was associated with a lesser threat of heart complaint. Another recent study set up that socially insulated aged grown-ups endured more habitual lung conditions and depressive symptoms compared to aged grown-ups with social support.

Feeling lonely can also impact memory. A study of further than 8,000 grown-ups aged than 65 set up that loneliness was linked to briskly cognitive decline.

Research also shows that being socially active can profit aged grown-ups. A study of further than 3,000 aged grown-ups set up that making new social connections was associated with bettered tone- reported physical and cerebral well- being. Being social may also help you reach your exercise pretensions. A 2019 study set up that aged grown-ups who had regular contact with musketeers and family were more physically active than those who did not.

Staying connected with others may help boost your mood and ameliorate your overall well- being. Stay in touch with family and musketeers in person or over the phone. Scheduling time each day to connect with others can help you maintain connections. Meet new people by taking a class to learn commodity new or hone a skill you formerly have.

Stress

Stress is a natural part of life and comes in numerous forms. Occasionally stress arises from delicate events or circumstances. Positive changes, like the birth of a grandchild or a creation, can beget stress too. Exploration shows that constant stress can change the brain, affect memory, and increase the threat of developing Alzheimer's or affiliated mania.

Aged grown-ups are at particular threat for stress and stress-related problems. A recent study examined how situations of the stress hormone cortisol change over time. Experimenters have set up that cortisol situations in a person's body increase steadily after middle age and that this age- related increase in stress may drive changes in the brain. A meta- analysis funded by the National Institute of Mental Health supports the notion that stress and anxiety rewire the brain in ways that can impact memory, decision- timber, and mood.

 Chancing ways to lower stress and increase emotional stability may support healthy aging. In an analysis of data from the Baltimore Longitudinal Study of Aging, scientists followed 2,000 actors for further than five decades, covering their moods and health. The data reveal that emotionally stable individualities lived on average three times longer than those who tended to be in a negative or anxious emotional state. Long- term stress also may contribute to or worsen a range of health problems, including digestive diseases, headaches, and sleep diseases.

You can help manage stress with contemplation ways, physical exertion, and sharing in conditioning you enjoy. Keeping a journal may also help you identify and challenge negative and harmful studies. Reach out to musketeers and family who can help you manage appreciatively.

Depression and overall mood

 Although depression is common in aged grown-ups, it can be delicate to fete. For some aged grown-ups with depression, sadness isn't their main symptom. Rather, they might feel numb or apathetic in conditioning and may not be as willing to talk about their passions. Depression not only affects internal health but also physical health. A review composition funded by the National Heart, Lung, and Blood Institute summarizes hundreds of studies from around the world showing that depression increases the threat of heart complaint and metabolic diseases. Research has also shown that intermittent depression is a threat factor for madness. In a study of further than 1,000 aged grown-ups, scientists set up a relationship between the number of depressive occurrences and an increased threat of developing Alzheimer's. The aged grown-up holding his head in his hands looks sad.

Although different than depression, which is a serious medical complaint, mood changes can also impact aging. A 2020 longitudinal study demonstrated a link between positive mood and better cognitive control. Farther studies are necessary to determine whether changes that ameliorate mood could ameliorate cognition. The way you suppose about aging can also make a difference. exploration shows that whether you hold negative or positive views about aging may impact your health as you age. Negative beliefs about aging may increase undesirable health issues, Alzheimer's complaint biomarkers, and cellular aging. Meanwhile, positive beliefs about aging may drop the threat of developing madness and rotundity.
Depression, indeed when severe, can be treated. As soon as you begin noticing signs, it's important to get estimated by a healthcare professional. In addition to deep sadness or impassiveness, lack of sleep and loss of appetite are also common symptoms of depression in aged adults. However, start by making an appointment to see your croaker or healthcare provider, if you suppose you or a loved one may have depression.

Rest conditioning and pursuits

Your favorite conditioning aren't only delightful they may also be good for your health. Exploration shows that people who share in pursuits and social and rest conditioning may be at lower threat for some health problems. For illustration, one study set up that participation in a community chorus program for aged grown-ups reduced loneliness and increased interest in life. Another study showed that aged grown-ups who spent at least an hour reading or engaged in other pursuits had a dropped threat of madness compared to those who spent lower than 30 twinkles a day on pursuits. Grandmother playing a game with her granddaughter

exploration on music, theater, cotillion , creative jotting, and other participatory trades shows pledge for perfecting aged grown-ups ' quality of life and well- being, from better cognitive function, memory, and tone- regard to reduced stress and increased social commerce. Indeed pursuits as simple as taking care of a pet can ameliorate your health. According to a 2020 study, pet power (or regular contact with faves) was associated with better cognitive function, and in some cases, better physical function.

Look for openings to share in conditioning. Get out and about by going to a sporting event, trying a new eatery, or visiting a gallery. Learn how to cook or play a musical instrument. Consider volunteering at an academy, library, or sanitarium to come more active in your community.

Taking care of your cognitive health

Cognition — the capability to suppose, learn, and flash back — frequently changes as we progress. Although some people develop Alzheimer's or other types of madness, numerous aged grown-ups witness more modest changes in memory and thinking. Exploration shows that healthy eating, staying active, and learning new chops may help keep aged grown-ups cognitively healthy.

How different factors affect cognitive health

Still, data from an NIH study with 3, 000 actors show else, if you suppose your diurnal choices do n't make a difference. Experimenters scored actors on five healthy life factors, all of which have important health benefits

- v At least 150 twinkles per week of moderate- to vigorous- intensity physical exertion
- v Not smoking
- v Not drinking heavily
- v A high- quality, Mediterranean- style diet
- v Engagement in mentally stimulating conditioning, similar as reading, writing letters, and playing games

The findings show that making these small, diurnal changes can add up to significant health benefits. Those who followed at least four of these healthy life actions had a 60 lower threat of developing Alzheimer's. Indeed rehearsing just two or three conditioning lowered the threat by 37. While results from experimental studies similar as this bone cannot prove cause and effect, they point to how a combination of adjustable actions may alleviate Alzheimer's threat and identify promising avenues to be tested in clinical trials.

How cognitive training affects health issues

Numerous brain training programs are retailed to the public to ameliorate cognition. Although some of these computer or smartphone- grounded interventions show pledge, so far there's no conclusive substantiation that these operations are salutary. But there's some substantiation that exercising your brain by learning a new skill can ameliorate memory function. A study of grown-ups 60 and aged showed that sustained engagement in cognitively demanding, new exertion enhanced memory function.

 Taking care of your physical, internal, and cognitive health is important for healthy aging. Indeed making small changes in your diurnal life can help you live longer and more. In general, you can support your physical health by staying active, eating and sleeping well, and going to the croaker regularly. Take care of your internal health by interacting with family and musketeers, trying to stay positive, and sharing in conditioning you enjoy. Taking way to achieve better physical and internal health may reduce your threat for Alzheimer's and affiliated mania as you age.

As we progress, it's important to maintain a healthy life to continue enjoying an active, fulfilled life. You can do this by fastening on habits similar as regular exercise, proper nutrition, and staying socially active.

Stay socially active with musketeers and family

Remaining socially connected as you get aged is extremely important to maintain your physical and internal health. People who are engaged in further social commerce are generally healthier individualities. Social commerce brings positive passions and decreases stress. Seniors who are more socially active also have lower rates of Alzheimer's.

One way to stay active socially is to try to share in group conditioning. Getting out of the house to have a healthy mess, or taking a walk with a friend, are fantastic ways to maintain connections and gemütlichkeit. Small group exercise classes will help you stick to an exercise program and produce a sense of fellowship.

Avoid Injuries

Make sure to exercise to stay healthy – and be careful not get injured. As we progress, our bodies suffer certain degenerative changes and plainness changes that make the senior further prone to injury during exercise. Balance may deteriorate and some of the specifics that we may be on can affect our exercise performance. Use lighter weights for delicate body corridor (shoulders) and avoid high- threat exercises. Make sure not to do the same movement too frequently, to avoid overuse injuries and avoid military-suchlike exercise training.

Start swimming

Incipiently, swimming is good exercise for seniors. It gets the heart rate over and is gentle on an arthritic body. Swimming is a great mood supporter to ward off depression, especially if the pool is outside and the sun is out.
Be Apprehensive of slower metabolism
 Unfortunately, as we progress, a braked metabolism, hormonal changes, and dropped muscle mass can lead to weight gain. Medical conditions can beget attempts at weight loss to be slow and taking specifics similar as antidepressants or corticosteroids may present a fresh challenge.
 You might not be exercising as constantly or as intensively as you need to for weight loss. However, you can take way

towards your thing by adding simple changes to your exercise routine, if you want to lose weight. For illustration, add a grade while you're using the routine, alternate walking or running pets, or try a cotillion class.

Try Yoga and Contemplation

Studies have set up that people who run, weight train, and cotillion have a lower threat of developing madness than people who aren't physically active at all. But if you can't take part in vigorous exertion, there's another option. A daily routine of yoga and contemplation may strengthen thinking chops and help to stave off aging- related internal decline.

One study compared people who took part in yoga with a group doing internal exercises as part of a brain- training program. The yoga actors spent an hour each week learning Kundalini yoga, which involves breathing exercises and contemplation, as well as movement and acts. The experimenters chose this form of yoga largely because people who are out of shape or new to yoga generally find it easy to complete the classes.

The yoga group also was tutored a type of contemplation known as Kirtan Kriya, which involves repeating a mantra and cutlet movements and asked to meditate in this way for 15 twinkles every day.

After 12 weeks, those who had rehearsed yoga and contemplation showed advancements in their moods and scored lower on a scale for implicit depression than the brain-training group. They also did better on a test of visuospatial memory, a type of flashing back that's important for balance, depth perception, and the capability to fete objects and navigate the world. In reviewing the brain reviews, experimenters set up those who had rehearsed yoga had developed more communication between corridor of the brain that control attention, suggesting a lesser capability now to concentrate and multitask.

CHAPTER TWO

HOW TO Ameliorate YOUR HEALTH

HEALTH & WELL- BEING

We impact our health through what we eat. Bread is embedded in our diurnal routine, making it the natural choice for a gut-friendly diet. Its filaments feed the good bacteria that are formerly present in one's gut, helping them thrive and transferring a ripple of well- being throughout the body and mind.

 Although chuck is embedded in simplicity, incinerating Happy Gut loaves of chuck is an art to master and wisdom to perfect. With over 100 times of moxie in bakery products at Puratos we noway stop exploring, allowing, and instituting, offering results that allow cookers to accessibly make the most infectious pieces of chuck with gut health benefits.

The bakery products in Puratos ' Happy Gut range all contain gut health- promoting composites, similar as specific types of filaments, which can help consumers ' gut health status.

Aware African mama with cute funny sprat son doing yoga exercise at home, the calm black mama and mixed race little girl sitting in lotus disguise on the settee together, mute tutoring the child to meditate

Digestive Health

The gastrointestinal tract of the digestive system is regularly exposed to food patches, environmental poisons, and pathogens. Maintaining a strong digestive system is essential for optimal health.

On a charge to help the mortal body gain the nutrition it needs to survive and thrive, the gastrointestinal(GI) tract of the digestive system is regularly exposed to food patches, environmental manures, and implicit pathogens. Maintaining a strong and healthy digestive system is crucial for promoting nutrient immersion, fostering a robust and different microbiome, and supporting general well- being and GI health.

Humans aren't always suitable to set their digestive systems up for success. In 2010, digestive conditions redounded in48.3 million visits to office- grounded healthcare providers, sanitarium inpatient conventions, and exigency departments across the UnitedStates.1- 2 A large maturity of these cases had digestive conditions as the primary opinion during their visit.1

Diet and GI Health

The types of foods people eat have a large impact on seditious status in the GI tract.3 For illustration, phytonutrients from factory- grounded foods and omega- 3 adipose acids in the diet are linked to healthy seditious responses in the GI tract.3 Phytonutrients from shops also support digestive health by modifying microbial populations in the microbiome and promoting intestinal hedgeintegrity.

Foods grandly in fiber are also important for a healthy GI tract. This is because bacteria that live in the GI tract break down fiber through turmoil, adding the product of short- chain adipose acids (SCFAs), like butyrate. Butyrate is associated with health goods in the body similar as guarding the blood-brain hedge, supporting intestinal health, and protection against antibioticexposure.

Fiber can be either water- undoable and less fermented or water-answerable and more fermented. Common sources of fiber include;

    v Vegetables
    v Legumes and seeds
    v Fruits
    v Whole grains

Diets with advanced quantities of fiber from shops contribute to plushly different microbiomes and increased situations of SFCA product in theintestine.10- 11 adding fiber consumption also supports intestinal health by adding bulk and relieving constipation.

Stress and GI Health

Increased stress can lead to redundant product of the stress hormone cortisol, which in turn can negatively affect the digestive system. This is because the " fight or flight " response to stress, quantified by changing cortisol situations, prioritizes blood inflow to the heart and brain, temporarily immolating lower vital organs like those in the digestive system. Historically, this diversion was necessary for a state of exigency when the cortisol shaft was warranted. Numerous ultramodern- day humans, however, experience habitual activation of the "fight or flight" response as a result of boosted cortisol situations from everyday stress. therefore, these same humans constantly witness the mischievous digestive goods of " fight or flight, " indeed when there's no exigency driving the response. These stressful cases have shown an capability to negatively impact the microbial populations in the lowerGI.

The Microbiome and GI Health

The healthy gut microbiome is a foundational part of digestive health. The microbiome is the massive population of microorganisms that live in the mortal body, like bacteria. Scientific substantiation makes significant connections between microbiome diversity, diet, and physiological goods – good and bad. For illustration, poor microbiome health is linked to increased situations of seditious cytokines.

The mortal microbiome begins to develop in immaturity. After birth and during early development, exposure to new energy sources from food and the external terrain shapes the content of the microbiome until a youthful child's microbiome reaches " adult status. " numerous factors may affect the content and diversity of the mortal microbiome antibiotic use, dragged tradition medicine use, salutary changes, gastrointestinal illness, development of habitual conditions, moving to a new country, short term trip, and indeed the stressful vacationseason.17- 24

Antibiotics & GI Health

Antibiotics can be mischievous to GI health by negatively impacting the growth of helpful microbiota, lowering biodiversity and dismembering the product of metabolic derivations from phytonutrients, compromising intestinal hedge integrity(conceivably leading to dense gut), and favoring the growth of opportunistic pathogens. Antibiotic-affiliated GI damage can be especially common in the senior, as they're one of the most generally specified specifics for this age group.29 fresh tradition specifics, similar as proton pump impediments and antipsychotics affect in a lower diversity of the microbiome.

GI Dysbiosis

GI dysbiosis can do when the balance of the intestinal terrain becomes disintegrated by stress, poor diet, limited physical exertion, or antibiotic overuse or abuse. This can be microbial population dependent where a person is out of the normal range of bacteria proportions(too numerous of some microbes and/ or too many salutary microbes).25 Whether because of genetics, early colonization, life, or other factors, GI dysbiosis is associated with a myriad of health conditions similar as Mood diseases(anxiety and depression).
Dense gut a condition characterized by weakened junctions between epithelial cells
 Nutrient deficiencies
 Phytonutrients and the Microbiome
For the utmost part, phytonutrients from factory foods circumvent chemical breakdown in the gut until they reach the

lower GI tract, allowing them to interact with the microbiota living there. Bacteria also break down these phytonutrients into metabolites small enough to also be absorbed through enterocytes and travel through the rotation.

Specific phytonutrients are uniquely suitable to support microbiota growth, which is associated with salutary goods, like perfecting intestinal hedgeintegrity. Phytonutrients can also impact microbial diversity in the GI tract by both enhancing and reducing bacterial populations. Microbial populations that profit from phytonutrient support include;

v Lactobacilli
v Bifidobacteria
v *Akkermansia muciniphilia*
v *Facalibacterium prausnitzii*

A study set up that a mama's metabolic status may impact the diversity of HMO composition in her breastmilk, which may affect the growth ofa.

Collinsonia Root for Digestive Health

Collinsonia Canadensis (Collinsonia; gravestone root) is a imperishable factory native to eastern North America with a rich history of traditional use.

Chlorella vulgaris and microalgae in general are bitsy but important sources of nutrition, including macronutrients, micronutrients, and phytonutrients.

Berberine for Gut and Metabolic Health

Berberine is a natural substance with antimicrobial goods, set up in Phellodendron dinghy, golden seal, Oregon grape, and numerous other sauces.
 What You Can Do to Maintain Your Health
A lot of factors play a part in staying healthy. In turn, good health can drop your threat of developing certain conditions. These include heart complaint, stroke, some cancers, and injuries.

Path to bettered health

Eat healthily.
What you eat is nearly linked to your health. Balanced nutrition has numerous benefits. By making healthier food choices, you can help or treat some conditions. These include heart complaint, stroke, and diabetes. A healthy diet can help you lose weight and lower your cholesterol, as well.
Get regular exercise.
Exercise can help heart complaint, stroke, diabetes, and colon cancer. It can help treat depression, osteoporosis, and high blood pressure. People who exercise also get injured less frequently. Routine exercise can make you feel more and keep your weight under control. Try to be active for 30 to 60 twinkles about 5 times a week. Flash back, any quantum of exercise is better than none.

Lose weight if you're fat.

Numerous Americans are fat. Carrying too important weight increases your threat for several health conditions. These include;

      v high blood pressure
      v high cholesterol
      v type 2 diabetes
      v heart complaint
      v stroke
      v some cancers
      v gallbladder complaint

Being fat also can lead to weight- related injuries. A common problem is an arthritis in the weight- bearing joints, similar as your chine, hips, or knees. There are several affects you can try to help you lose weight and keep it off.

Cover your skin.

Sun exposure is linked to skin cancer. This is the most common type of cancer that's affecting us. It's stylish to limit your time spent in the sun. Be sure to wear defensive apparel and headdresses when you're outdoors. Use sunscreen time-round on exposed skin, like your face and hands. It protects your skin and helps help skin cancer. Choose a broad-diapason sunscreen that blocks both UVA and UVB shafts. Don't sunbathe or use tanning cells.

Practice safe coitus.

Safe coitus is good for your emotional and physical health. The safest form of coitus is between 2 people who only have coitus with each other. Use protection to help sexually transmitted conditions (STDs). Condoms are the most effective form of forestallment. Talk to your croaker
 If you need to be tested for STDs.

Do n't bank or use tobacco.

Smoking and tobacco use are dangerous habits. They can beget heart complaint and mouth, throat, or lung cancer.They also are leading factors of emphysema and habitual obstructive pulmonary complaint (COPD). The sooner you quit, the better.
Limit how important alcohol you drink.
Men should have no further than 2 drinks a day. Women should have no further than 1 drink a day. One drink is equal to 12 ounces of beer, 5 ounces of wine, or1.5 ounces of liquor. Too important alcohol can damage your liver. It can beget some cancers, similar as throat, liver, or pancreas cancer. Alcohol abuse also contributes to deaths from auto smashups, murders, and self-murders.
 You need to make time for bone health. Bone cancer is a leading cause of death for women. Men can get bone cancer, too. Talk to your croaker about when you should start getting mammograms. You may need to start screening beforehand if

you have threat factors, similar as a family history. One way to descry bone cancer is to do a yearly tone- test.

Women should get routine pap smears, as well. Women aged 21 to 65 should get tested every 3 times. This may differ if you have certain conditions.

Keep a list of current drugs you take. You also should stay up to date on shots, including getting an periodic flu shot. Grown-ups need a Td supporter every 10 times. Your croaker may substitute it with Tdap. This also protects against whooping cough (pertussis). Women who are pregnant need the Tdap vaccine. People who are in close contact with babies should get it, as well.

CHAPTER THREE

WHAT ARE THE Conditions FOR HEALTHY LIFE

At Healthfully, we strive to deliver objective content that's accurate and over- to- date. Our platoon periodically reviews papers to insure happy quality. The sources cited below correspond of substantiation from peer- reviewed journals, prominent medical associations, academic associations, and government data.

The Conditions for a Healthy Life

v Eat Healthy Food

v Get Physical Exercise
v Steer Clear
v Take preventative Measures

Living life involves knowledge about introductory survival chops paired with making connections to people who help you get your requirements met. In themid-1900s, humanistic psychologist Abraham Maslow linked his proposition of the introductory requirements for successful mortal progression, supposed the" scale of requirements." Within this scale, the first and most important requirements included introductory survival, or physiological requirements, followed by safety and belonging. Although a proposition, the scale, paired with medical advancement, is useful as a guideline for healthy living and precluding controllable conditions.

Eat Healthy Food

Eat nutritional foods as they're essential to physiological survival. Skipping refection's, eating massive portions, or binge eating and consuming high- fat or high- calorie refection's limits your energy and nutrient immersion. Food is the introductory energy of life. Start with the introductory food groups, like fruits and vegetables, whole grains, dairy, and meat.
Eat raw or steamed vegetables rather of fried or microwaved particulars. Use the USDA Food Guide Aggregate as a guideline for food servings and mess planning.
Eat Nutritional foods as they're essential to physiological survival.

Get Physical Exercise

A Healthy Food Plan for Breakfast, Lunch, regale & Snacks. Physical exertion is important in reducing your threat of rotundity, diabetes, and heart complaint. It also stimulates your internal heartiness by adding brain chemicals involved in regulating your mood, sleep, and appetite. The American Heart Association advises exercising for at least 30 twinkles a day by walking, joining a fitness class, or engaging in yard work. For every hour you engage in exercise, like walking, you may add two hours to your life.

It can be delicate to fit exercise into your diurnal routine but try walking around your neighborhood rather of watching a 30-nanosecond TV show. Get your family involved in the exercise to make it delightful or ask musketeers to join you in getting healthier.
Physical exertion is important in reducing your threat of rotundity, diabetes, and heart complaint.
Get your family involved in an exercise to make it delightful or ask musketeers to join you in getting healthier.

Steer Clear

Smoking, drinking inordinate quantities of alcohol, and lawless medicine use like cocaine or marijuana increase your threat of liver, lung, and heart diseases. Steer clear of medicine use altogether and find support to help you stop smoking. Drink no further than seven alcoholic potables a week if you're womanish or if you're manly.

Smoking, drinking inordinate quantities of alcohol, and lawless medicine use like cocaine or marijuana increase your threat of liver, lung, and heart diseases.
Seek comforting or a support group if you drink to excess.
Take preventative Measures
How to make Muscle without Creating

With the arrival of ultramodern drug, there are plenitude of options for monthly health wireworks to catch early signs of complaint. Set up periodic physical health visits so your croaker can give the necessary interventions.
Take preventives in your diurnal life by washing your hands before handling food, after using the bathroom, and in dealing with people in a medical setting. Use prophylactics before engaging in sexual contact and limit sexual mates. Place sunscreen on your body to cover your skin from sun damage. Avoid distractions while driving like talking on the cell phone. Don't drink alcohol or use medicines and drive. Cover yourself from unintended injury from auto accidents by wearing a seat belt.
With the arrival of ultramodern drug, there are plenitude of options for monthly health wireworks to catch early signs of complaint.
Take preventives in your diurnal life by washing your hands before handling food, after using the bathroom, and in dealing with people in a medical setting.

A Balanced Life

Manage your diurnal stress by taking the time to relax after a long day. Go to a quiet room or hear to calming music. Join a yoga or contemplation class to learn breathing and relaxation ways. Keep in touch with your loved bones and seek support from those you're closest to as a means of managing with stress.

Take the time to fraternize on the weekends to nurture your introductory need to connect with others in society. Find a healthy balance between work, connections, home, and rest time.

Manage your diurnal stress by taking the time to relax after a long day.

Take the time to fraternize on the weekends to nurture your introductory need to connect with others in society.

What does fact- check mean?

Healthfully , we strive to deliver objective content that's accurate and over- to- date. Our platoon periodically reviews papers to ensure happy quality. The sources cited below correspond to substantiation from peer- reviewed journals, prominent medical associations, academic associations, and government data.

Essential for a Healthy Diet

Eating healthy doesn't have to taste bland. However, try opting foods that are analogous to those you presently eat, If you're transitioning into a healthy diet. Begin by replacing unhealthy, empty calories with nutrient-rich constituents. Eat moderate portions of food within your sweet input pretensions. As you feel comfortable eating healthy, increase your input of raw and picked foods.

Breakfast

Try a healthy interpretation of bagels and lox by eating a whole- grain bagel rather of one made with refined white flour. Whole grains give salutary fiber essential for a healthy digestive system, according to the Mayo Clinic 1. Use low- fat non-dairy cream rubbish rather of the full- fat variety and blend in some knaveries. Add Non-genetically modified salmon for essential adipose acids, which help reduce inflammation and help degenerative conditions.
 Try a healthy interpretation of bagels and lox by eating a whole- grain bagel rather of one made with refined white flour.

Lunch

For lunch, eat a whole- grain serape or sandwich. Avoid reused deli flesh for healthy lunches; rather, use organic deli meat or an organic, soy- grounded meat volition. In the sandwich or serape, place a variety of vegetables, similar as

> v sprouts
> v dark leafy flora
> v avocado
> v tomato
> v onion

Spread hummus on the chuck or serape in place of mayonnaise or other seasonings. rather than eating French feasts or chips on the side, have a small salad or broth-grounded haze.

For lunch, eat a whole- grain serape or sandwich.

Regale

Regale can correspond of a serving of protein like organic funk, meat, and tempeh. Tempeh, made from fermented soybeans, contains probiotics that act as "friendly" bacteria, helping alleviate dangerous bacteria in your bowel. This is especially helpful if you take antibiotics, which kill both dangerous and helpful bacteria. Along with protein, have a large helping of grilled or fumed vegetables and a small side of whole grains. Some vegetable ideas are grilled asparagus, fumed artichoke, ignited sweet potato, or sauteed spinach or kale. Add a splash of olive oil painting, ocean swab, and fresh bomb juice to season your vegetables.

Regale can correspond of a serving of protein like organic funk, meat, tempeh, or seitan.

Tempeh, made from fermented soybeans, contains probiotics that act as " friendly " bacteria, helping alleviate dangerous bacteria in your bowel.

Replace sticky, fried snacks with foods that will give nutrition and energy. Carrot sticks with natural nut adulation that doesn't contain incompletely hydrogenated canvases . Add raisins for a good source of iron.

Replace sticky, fried snacks with foods that will give nutrition and energy.

Eat celery or carrot sticks with natural nut adulation that doesn't contain incompletely hydrogenated canvases.

Health and fitness magazines give a wide variety of papers that make claims to increase your muscle mass with the use of creatine. Creatine, a gratuitous salutary element set up in meat and fish, is used as a supplement by athletes to enhance exercise performance. While creatine is perceived as fairly safe, the American College of Sports Medicine notes that there is been little critical evaluation and exploration done to establish the positive and negative health impacts of this supplement. Adding your muscle mass is attainable without taking creatine.

Perform weighted emulsion exercises that work for multiple muscle groups at the same time like bench presses, lat pull-campo, syllables, and lunges. Mix with body weight emulsion exercises like drive- ups, pull- ups, and burpees.

Eat every three to four hours to fuel your exercises and aid in muscle recovery. Avoid reused foods. Consume foods in their whole form fastening on fruits, vegetables, spare proteins, and complex carbohydrates.

Get some rest. Take at least one rest day per week to allow muscles to recover from your exercises. Sleep eight hours per night to allow the release of growth hormones that help make muscle.

Drink 1 gallon of water per day to stay doused and support exertion. Drink enough water to replace your diurnal losses and drink further on days when temperature and moisture are high.

Tips

Lift heavy weights and keep your reiterations low. The last many reiterations should be veritably grueling .

Lifestyle Tips for A Healthy Limbic System

The limbic system represents the part of your brain devoted to the most introductory survival structures that cover and regulate feelings and reactive countries. Hitching pathways link the limbic system, located deep within your brain, to the hypothalamus, which controls thinking, geste and hormonal functions. The main limbic structures include the hippocampus, or memory center; the amygdala, or wrathfulness, anxiety, and stress center; and the limbic cortex which interconnects with the prefrontal cortex, which is responsible for logic and judgment. Your emotional heartiness is contingent upon a healthy limbic system and deterioration in this area of your brain can lead to out- of- control feelings like violence or rage, depression, and neurological decline.

Eat a nutrient-rich diet high in fruit, vegetables, and whole grains. Produce and grains are your main sources of natural vitamins, minerals, and antioxidants that cover your brain cells from dangerous motes. Several diurnal servings of fresh fruits, vegetables, and whole grains can help you maintain the chemicals produced in your brain, called neurotransmitters that are demanded to prompt a healthy limbic system.

Limit impregnated fats and replace them with omega- 3 adipose acids. Foods grandly in impregnated fats include red meat, fried foods, and whole dairy. redundant impregnated fats in your diet increase the threat of habitual neurodegenerative conditions like Alzheimer's. Omega- 3 adipose acids from foods like fish or nuts can cover your brain and help to keep your mood stabilized.

Stay connected to those you watch about and fraternize regularly. Emotional health is nurtured by the bonds created from connections. Nourish your feelings by visiting with family regularly, catching a movie with musketeers, or by sometimes forming new social connections.

Exercise regularly to stimulate your body and mind. Exercise helps to elevate mood and increase the product of neurotransmitters that help you sleep, suppose and feel. An authority of exercise for 20 to 30 twinkles, three to five times a week, can help maintain limbic system health.

The limbic system is naturally touched off by scents, and calming or amping aromas can help stimulate this part of your brain while also regulating your feelings.
Replace impregnated with unsaturated fat
Fats are important for good health and proper functioning of the body. Still, too much of it can negatively affect our weight and cardiovascular health. Different kinds of fats have different health goods, and some of these tips could help us keep the balance right
We should limit the consumption of total and logged fats (frequently coming from foods of beast origin), and fully avoid trans fats; reading the markers helps to identify the sources.
Eating fish 2- 3 times a week, with at least one serving of unctuous fish, will contribute to our right input of unsaturated fats.
When cooking, we should boil, foam or singe, rather than frying, remove the adipose part of the meat, and use vegetable canvases.

Drink plenitude of fluids

Grown-ups need to drink at least1.5 liters of fluid a day! Or further if it's veritably hot or they're physically active. Water is the stylish source, of course, and we can use valve or mineral water, foamy or non-sparkling, plain or seasoned. Fruit authorities, tea, soft drinks, milk, and other drinks, can all be okay- from time to time.

Reduce swab and sugar input
A high swab input can affect high blood pressure, and increase the threat of cardiovascular complaint. There are different ways to reduce swab in the diet

When shopping, we could choose products with lower sodium content.

When cooking, swab can be substituted with spices, adding the variety of flavors and tastes.

When eating, it helps not to have swab at the table, or at least not to add swab before tasting.

Sugar provides agreeableness and an seductive taste, but sticky foods and drinks are rich in energy and are stylish enjoyed in temperance, as an occasional treat. We could use fruits rather, indeed to candy our foods and drinks.

Eat regularly, control the portion size

Eating a variety of foods, regularly, and in the right quantities is the stylish formula for a healthy diet.

Skipping refections, especially breakfast, can lead to out- of-control hunger, frequently performing in helpless gluttony. Gorging between refections can help control hunger, but snacking shouldn't replace proper refections. For snacks, we could choose yogurt, a sprinkle of fresh or dried fruits or vegetables(like carrot sticks), unsalted nuts, or maybe some chuck with rubbish.

Paying attention to portion size will help us not to consume too numerous calories, and will allow us to eat all the foods we enjoy, without having to exclude any.

Cooking the right quantum makes it easier to not gormandize.

Some reasonable serving sizes are 100 g of meat; one medium piece of fruit; half a mug of raw pasta.

Using lower plates helps with lower servings.

Packaged foods, with calorie values on the pack, could prop portion control.

Still, we could partake a portion with a friend, If eating out.

CHAPTER FOUR

WHAT ARE THE BENEFITS OF EXERCISE TO YOUR BODY

Benefits of Physical exertion
Regular physical exertion is one of the most important affects you can do for your health. Being physically active can ameliorate your brain health, help manage weight, reduce the threat of complaint, strengthen bones and muscles, and ameliorate your capability to do everyday conditioning.
Grown-ups who sit less and do any quantum of moderate- to-vigorous physical exertion gain some health benefits. Only a many life choices have as large an impact on your health as physical exertion.
Everyone can witness the health benefits of physical exertion – age, capacities, race, shape, or size don't count.

Immediate Benefits

Some benefits of physical exertion on brain health be right after a session of moderate- to-vigorous physical exertion. Benefits include bettered thinking or cognition for children 6 to 13 times of age and reduced short- term passions of anxiety for grown-ups. Regular physical exertion can help keep your thinking, literacy, and judgment chops sharp as you age. It can also reduce your threat of depression and anxiety and help you sleep better.

Weight Management

Both eating patterns and physical exertion routines play a critical part in weight operation. You gain weight when you consume further calories through eating and drinking than the number of calories you burn, including those burned during physical exertion. To maintain your weight Work your way up to 150 twinkles a week of moderate physical exertion, which could include dancing or yard work. You could achieve the thing of 150 twinkles a week with 30 twinkles a day, 5 days a week.
People vary greatly in how important physical exertion they need for weight operation. You may need to be more active than others to reach or maintain a healthy weight.
To lose weight and keep it off You'll need a high quantum of physical exertion unless you also acclimate your eating patterns and reduce the number of calories you 're eating and drinking. Getting to and staying at a healthy weight requires both regular physical exertion and healthy eating.

Reduce Your Health threat

Hysterical of Getting Hurt?
The good news is that moderate physical exertion, similar as brisk walking, is generally safe for utmost people.

Cardiovascular Disease

Heart complaint and stroke are two leading causes of death in the United States. Getting at least 150 twinkles a week of moderate physical exertion can put you at a lower threat for these conditions. You can reduce your threat indeed further with further physical exertion. Regular physical exertion can also lower your blood pressure and ameliorate your cholesterol situations.
Type 2 Diabetes and Metabolic Pattern
Regular physical exertion can reduce your threat of developing type 2 diabetes and metabolic pattern. Metabolic pattern is some combination of too important fat around the midriff, high blood pressure, low high- viscosity lipoproteins (HDL) cholesterol, high triglycerides, or high blood sugar. People start to see benefits at situations from a physical exertion indeed without meeting the recommendations for 150 twinkles a week of moderate physical exertion. Fresh quantities of physical exertion feel to lower threat indeed more.
Some Cancers
Being physically active lowers your threat of developing several common cancers. Grown-ups who share in lesser

quantities of physical exertion have reduced pitfalls of developing cancers of the;

v Bladder
v bone
v Colon(proximal and distal)
v Endometrium
v Esophagus(adenocarcinoma)
v order
v Lung
v Stomach(cardia andnon-cardia adenocarcinoma)

 Still, getting regular physical exertion not only helps give you a better quality of life but also improves your physical fitness, if you're a cancer survivor.

Regular Physical exertion Helps Lower Your Cancer threat
Strengthen Your Bones and Muscles
A woman jogging in a demesne with her canine.
As you age, it's important to cover your bones, joints, and muscles – they support your body and help you move. Keeping bones, joints, and muscles healthy can help insure that you 're suitable to do your diurnal conditioning and be physically active.
Muscle- strengthening conditioning like lifting weights can help you increase or maintain your muscle mass and strength. This is important for aged grown-ups who witness reduced muscle mass and muscle strength with aging. Sluggishly adding the quantum of weight and number of reiterations you do as part of muscle- strengthening conditioning will give you indeed more benefits, no matter your age. Ameliorate Your Capability to do Daily Conditioning and help falls everyday conditioning include climbing stairs, grocery shopping, or playing with your grandchildren. Being unfit to do everyday conditioning is called a functional limitation. Physically active middle-aged or aged

grown-ups have a lower threat of functional limitations than inactive people.

For aged grown-ups, doing a variety of physical conditioning improves physical function and decreases the threat of cascade or injury from a fall. Include physical conditioning similar as calisthenics, muscle strengthening, and balance training. Multicomponent physical exertion can be done at home or in a community setting as part of a structured program.

Hipsterism fracture is a serious health condition that can affect from a fall. Breaking a hipsterism have life- changing negative goods, especially if you 're an aged grown-up. Physically active people have a lower threat of hipsterism fracture than inactive people.

Increase Your Chances of Living Longer

How important Physical exertion Do I Need?

See physical exertion recommendations for different groups, including;

- v Children age 3- 5.
- v Children and adolescents age 6- 17.
- v Grown-ups progressed 18- 64.
- v Grown-ups 65 and aged.
- v Grown-ups with habitual health conditions and disabilities.

Healthy pregnant and postpartum women.

An estimated 110,000 deaths per time could be averted if US grown-ups periods 40 and aged increased their moderate- to-vigorous physical exertion by a small quantum. Indeed 10 twinkles more a day would make a difference.

Taking further way a day also helps lower the threat of unseasonable death from all causes. For grown-ups youngish than 60, the threat of unseasonable death leveled off at about 8,000 to 10,000 way per day. For grown-ups 60 and aged, the

threat of unseasonable death leveled off at about 6,000 to 8,000 way per day.
Manage Chronic Health Conditions & Disabilities
Regular physical exertion can help people manage being habitual conditions and disabilities. For illustration, regular physical exertion can reduce pain and ameliorate function and quality of life for grown-ups with arthritis.
Help control blood sugar situations and lower the threat of heart complaint and whim-whams damage for people with type 2 diabetes.
Regular exercising routine is one of the surest paths to a longer and healthier life. It's recommended that grown-ups get at least 150 twinkles of exercise every week, but not indeed half of us do so. We can find stacks of defenses for procrastinating and not exercising, but then's a list of reasons why we should do so.

Establish a Healthy Routine

- To take advantage of spa class (and cost), you'll tend to make yourself go to the spa regularly. It becomes easy to establish a healthy routine with all the installations and classes at your fingertips! So flip that fiscal chain into a motivator, establish a routine and you'll produce a new healthy habit well worth the investment in no time.

Get Stress Relief

- Any form of exercise can act as a stress reliever. Physical exertion boosts the brain's product of endorphins, which simply makes us feel more physically and have a brighter emotional outlook overall. Exercise physically reduces pressure in both the body and the mind which can ameliorate your mood and the quality of your sleep.

- Gymnasiums are now filled with professional coaches on staff, they're all trained to help you achieve your fitness pretensions and to design exercise programs that fit your individual requirements in a fun and safe way. utmost spa staff are friendly and further than ready to show you proper exercise ways so that you do n't hurt yourself and to insure you get the most out of each exercise routine.
 Sample the Fitness Classes
- currently, gymnasiums have a huge selection of exercise classes and other fitness rudiments. This allows you to try new types of fitness trends to vary your routine. However, your body builds a type of muscle memory, and the earnings you make are incrementally dropped, if you do the same drill day in and day out.
 Access to Equipment
- One of the biggest advantages are the wide array of outfit available! It might be bogarting at first, but you 'll find friendly experts on hand to help you use it all. Trust us it's a lot simpler than it looks once you get the hang of it!
Sweat Together
-numerous people find fitness classes to be the most effective and delightful way to get a full- body drill. You can do everything from HIIT to CrossFit, and from boxing to yoga. There's generally a veritably energetic educator to help give you with some redundant energy and provocation. These classes are generally filled with regulars, so it's nice to see everyone in the inflow together or perhaps indeed make new musketeers!

Increased Energy situations

- One of the benefits of exercising is an increase in energy situations and enhanced mood, due to the release of natural, happy endorphins. However, you'll surely feel reenergized and ready for the day after a great drill!
 If you're looking for a redundant spring in your step.

Be Motivated

- You either love to exercise or have to drag yourself to get it done. However, heading to the spa and being around others who are in the same situation as you can be just the incitement and provocation you need to keep going, If you 're one of the ultimate. You might indeed find yourself converting into an exercise nut when you start heading to the spa on a further regular base, hitting your fitness pretensions and seeing results on the inside and out!
 You do n't need to do the absolute outside or try to keep up with the veritably buff- looking person working out hard on your first day. Take it slow and steady, which can avoid overstepping yourselves or getting hurt.
We've all heard it numerous times before-regular exercise is good for you, and it can help you lose weight. But if you're like numerous Americans, you're busy, you have a sedentary job, and you have not yet changed your exercise habits. The good news is that it's noway too late to start. You can start sluggishly, and find ways to fit further physical exertion into your life. To get the most benefit, you should try to get the recommended quantum of exercise for your age.However, the

lucre is that you'll feel more, help help or control numerous conditions, If you can do it.

What are the health benefits of exercise?

Regular exercise and physical exertion may

Help you control your weight. Along with diet, exercise plays an important part in controlling your weight and precluding rotundity. To maintain your weight, the calories you eat and drink must equal the energy you burn. To lose weight, you must use further calories than you eat and drink.

Reduce your threat of heart complaint. Exercise strengthens your heart and improves your rotation. The increased blood inflow raises the oxygen situations body. This helps lower your threat of heart conditions similar as high cholesterol, coronary roadway complaint, and heart attack. Regular exercise can also lower your blood pressure and triglyceride situations.

CHAPTER FIVE

HOW TO AVOID DIGESTIVE ISSUES

From disturbing gas to uncomfortable heartburn, everyone has digestive problems from time to time. The good news is there are some simple results for numerous of your troubles. Learn about what causes your discomfort, how to help and manage digestive problems, what questions to ask your druggist, and when to see a croaker
Your digestive system is made up of numerous organs.
The Digestive System
How does the digestive system work?
It may feel like digestion only happens in your stomach, but it's a long process that involves numerous organs. Together they form the digestive tract.
Digestion begins in your mouth, where slaver starts to break down food when you bite. When you swallow, your masticated food moves to your esophagus, a tube that connects your throat to your stomach. Muscles in the esophagus push the food down to a stopcock at the bottom of your esophagus, which opens to let food into the stomach.
Your stomach breaks food down using stomach acids. also the food moves into the small intestine. There, digestive authorities from several organs, like your pancreas and gallbladder, break down the food more, and nutrients are absorbed. What's left goes through your large intestine. The large intestine absorbs water. The waste also moves out of your body through the rectum and anus.
 Digestive problems can be anywhere along the way.

Gas and Bloating

Bloating and passing gas can be uncomfortable and disturbing. Then's what you need to know.

What's gas?

Gas is a normal part of healthy digestion. Air that's in your digestive tract is either released through your mouth as a belch or through your anus as gas. You generally pass gas 13 to 21 times a day.
What causes gas?
Gas is created when you swallow air, similar as when you eat and drink. But it's also a derivate of the breakdown of food. Some foods beget further gas than others. You may also be more sensitive to particular foods and may have further gas when you eat them.
Which foods beget gas?
You 've presumably noticed you feel gaseous after eating certain foods. Cut back on the common lawbreakers

- v Apples
- v Asparagus
- v sap
- v Broccoli
- v Brussels sprouts
- v Cabbage
- v Cauliflower
- v Milk and dairy products
- v Mushrooms

v Onions
v Peaches
v Pears
v Prunes
v Wheat

What causes bloating?

When gas builds up in your stomach and bowel, you may have to bloat – lump in your belly and a feeling of wholeness. It may be to you more frequently if you have
A stomach infection
perverse bowel pattern(IBS). This digestive condition causes stomach pain, cramping, and diarrhea or constipation.
Celiac complaint. When people with this condition eat gluten, their bodies produce antibodies that attack the intestinal filling.
Hormonal changes that be around women's ages
Constipation
While bloating is generally just uncomfortable, it can occasionally beget pain in your belly or sides.
How can I reduce gas and bloating?
Diet and life changes can make a big difference
Cut back on adipose foods.
Avoid effervescent drinks.
Eat and drink sluggishly.
Quit smoking.
Do n't bite goo.
Exercise more.
Avoid foods that beget gas.
Avoid sweeteners that beget gas similar as fructose and sorbitol. They're frequently set up in delicacies, biting goo, energy bars, and low- carb foods.
What OTC drugs treat redundant gas?

still, untoward drug may help, If you have a lot of gas or are veritably uncomfortable.

Lactase supplements. However, taking these tablets or drops just before you eat will help you digest lactose(the main sugar in dairy foods) and reduce gas, If dairy is causing your problems. nascence- galactosidase. This digestive aid comes as liquid or tablets. You take it before you eat to help your body break down the complex carbs or sugars that beget gas, similar as those set up in sap, broccoli, and cabbage. Caution People with the inheritable condition galactosemia should avoid it. It may also intrude with some diabetes medicines like acarbose(Precose) or miglitol(Glyset). still, talk to your croaker

or druggist before taking this aid, If you take drug for diabetes.

Simethicone(Mylicon). Taking these liquids or tablets can relieve the uncomfortable bloating and pain from gas.

Probiotics. These supplements contain" friendly" bacteria that can help digestion. In addition to tablets and maquillages you sprinkle on your food, foods like yogurt, kefir, and sauerkraut contain probiotics.

Heartburn/ GERD

What's heartburn?

Heartburn, occasionally called acid indigestion, is a painful, burning feeling in the middle of your casket or the upper part of your stomach. The pain, which can also spread to your neck, jaw, or arms, can last just a many twinkles or stick with you for hours.

What causes heartburn?

There's a muscle at the entrance of your stomach, called the lower esophageal sphincter (LES), that acts like a gate It opens to let food move from your esophagus to your stomach, and it shuts to stop food and acid from coming back out.

When the LES opens too frequently or is n't tight enough, stomach acid can rise into the esophagus and beget a burning feeling.

What triggers heartburn?

Alarms vary from person to person, but you may be more likely to get heartburn when you gormandize
Eat racy, adipose, acidic, or slithery foods
Consume caffeine or alcohol.

Who gets heartburn?

Some people have an advanced threat of heartburn, including those who are;

· Smokers
· fat
· Pregnant

Have a hiatal hernia, where the stomach bulges up into the casket through an opening in the diaphragm

How should I change my diet to avoid heartburn?

You might have noticed that your heartburn gets worse when you eat or drink certain effects. Then are a many that can spark heartburn

Alcohol
Chocolate
Coffee
Adipose or fried foods
slithery foods
Onions
Oranges, failures, and other citrus fruits and authorities
ginger, hot gravies, and salad dressings
Peppermint
Sodas and other gamesome drinks
Spicy foods
Tomatoes and tomato sauce
Big refections can also set off heartburn. rather of eating three big refections a day, try to eat several small refections throughout the day.
What differently can I do to help heartburn?

Then are a many way to try lose weight if you're fat. redundant pounds put pressure on your stomach, forcing further acid up into your esophagus.
Wear loose apparel. Tight clothes that press on your stomach can spark heartburn.
Still, quit, If you bomb. Cigarette bank relaxes the muscle that prevents acid from backing up into the esophagus. It also may increase how important acid your stomach makes.
Check your drugs. Regular use ofanti-inflammatory and pain drugs (other than acetaminophen) contributes to heartburn.
Avoid high- impact exercise.

If heartburn bothers you at night
Eat a light regale and avoid foods that spark your heartburn.
Do n't lie down for at least 2 to 3 hours after you eat.
Use blocks or books to raise the head of your bed by 4- 6 elevation. Or put a froth wedge under your mattress at the head of the bed. Sleeping at an angle will help stop acid from backing up into your esophagus.

Can exercise cause heartburn?

Exercise has further than many health benefits. Among them is weight loss, which can help you avoid getting heartburn in the first place if you're fat. But some types of exercise can spark the burning sensation. You'll be less likely to reach for your heartburn drug if you avoid crunches and reversed acts in yoga. You may need to find druthers to high- impact exercises. For illustration, bike or swim rather of going for a run.

What's GERD?

Everyone has heartburn from time to time. But when you have it constantly (at least twice a week for a many weeks), or when it begins to intrude with your diurnal life or damage your esophagus, your croaker may tell you that you have a long-term condition called gastroesophageal influx complaint, or GERD. It's also known as acid influx complaint. Heartburn is the most common symptom of GERD.

What are the other symptoms of GERD?
Besides the frequent burning in your casket, you might also have symptoms like;

· Bad breath or a sour taste in your mouth or in the reverse of your throat
· Breathing problems
· Coughing
· Feeling like you lump the reverse of your throat
· Coarse or raspy voice
· Nausea
· delicate or painful swallowing
· Sore throat
· Tooth decay
· Vomiting

Is it GERD or commodity differently?

Frequent heartburn is a symptom of GERD. It's important to get help if you have heartburn constantly so you can avoid complications from GERD and uncover any other problems. Call your croaker or make an appointment with a gastroenterologist, who specializes in digestive ails. Numerous of the symptoms of heartburn sound like a heart attack.

What are the complications of frequent heartburn and GERD?

Over time, heartburn that is n't treated or controlled well by life changes or drug may beget serious problems, including

Breathing problems like asthma, darkness choking, and repeated pneumonia

Changes in the cells that line the esophagus, called Barrett's esophagus. This can lead to cancer of the esophagus.
Painful inflammation of the esophagus called esophagitis
Narrowing of the esophagus, called an esophageal stricture. This can beget problems swallowing.
What drugs can I take to treat heartburn?

Several types of over-the-counter (OTC) and tradition drugs can help with heartburn. Your croaker
or druggist can help you find the bone
that's right for you.

Antacids

Soothe occasional, mild heartburn with an antacid that contains calcium carbonate or magnesium. They help neutralize stomach acid. Some help acid influx. Those that contain magnesium may also help heal stomach ulcers. They come in liquids and capsules and are fast- amusement.
Antacids can beget constipation and diarrhea. Look for brands that contain calcium carbonate, magnesium hydroxide, and aluminum hydroxide to reduce these side goods. Do n't take antacids with magnesium if you have habitual order complaint. Some antacids have a lot of swab, so you should take them only for occasional heartburn.

H2 Blockers
H2 blockers help relieve and help occasional heartburn by lowering the quantum of acid your stomach makes. Though they do n't work as presto as antacids, their goods last longer. Your croaker

may tell you to take an antacid and an H2 blocker together. H2 blockers are for short- term use – lower than 2 weeks. You can take them before your refections to help heartburn, or at bedtime. They come in liquids and capsules. All H2 blockers work about the same. So if one does n't help with your heartburn, switching to a different bone is n't likely to help. Switching to an advanced- cure tradition interpretation of the medicine might help, however. Talk to your croaker
If over-the-counter H2 blockers are not working for you.
Some H2 blockers can intrude with other medicines, including;

    v Anti-seizure drugs
    v Blood thinners
    v Medicines for heart meter problems

What are the side goods of H2 blockers?

The most common side goods are mild and include;

    v Constipation
    v Diarrhea
    v Headache
    v Nausea or puking
    v Proton- Pump Impediments(PPIs)

What are PPIs?

 PPIs are used to help frequent heartburn that happens further than twice a week. They work by lowering the quantum of acid your stomach makes. Frequently, they work better than H2 blockers. You also can take these medicines for a longer period than H2 blockers.
PPIs are available over the counter and by tradition. But if you have GERD, you may need tradition- strength drug.

How do you take PPIs?

You need to take PPIs once a day on an empty stomach so they 'll work stylish. Generally you 'll take the drug every morning, about 30 to 60 twinkles before you eat breakfast, to control stomach acid. Before taking the PPI called omeprazole (Prilosec OTC) if you take clopidogrel(Plavix), a medicine used to help heart attacks and strokes. Taking the two medicines may make clopidogrel less effective.

What are the side goods of PPIs?

The most common side goods are mild and include

    v Diarrhea

v Headache
v Nausea and puking
v Stomach pain

 PPIs may also raise your chances of getting order complaint, and fractures of the hipsterism, wrist, and spin, and may lead to low magnesium situations. The threat is loftiest in people who take high cure PPIs for a time or further.

Prokinetics

Prokinetics help your stomach empty briskly, so you have lower acid left before. Generally you take this drug before refections and at bedtime. Prokinetics are vended only by tradition.
What are the side goods of prokinetics?
Prokinetics can have more serious side goods than PPIs or H2 blockers. These include;

v Anxiety
v Depression
v Diarrhea
v Doziness
v Fatigue
v huffiness
v Nausea

your drugs beget side goods you ca n't tolerate, or you have other complications, If your heartburn is n't getting better. It's rare to need surgery for heartburn.

still, you can take one of these tests to find out what is causing the problem

If drug and life changes do n't control your heartburn.

pH test. This measures the acidity of your esophagus. The croaker will either attach a small detector to your esophagus or place a thin tube down your esophagus.

BariumX-ray. You 'll drink a liquid that fleeces the inside of your digestive tract. alsoX-rays are taken, which will allow your croaker to see the figure of your digestive system.

When is heartburn an exigency?

Heartburn is generally a minor problem that goes down over time. But if you also have other symptoms, it could be a sign that commodity more serious is wrong. Call your croaker or go to the exigency room if it hurts to swallow.

You feel like you're choking.

You have black, sojourn- looking bowel movements.

Your mouth or throat hurts when you eat.

You have difficulty swallowing foods

Your voice is coarse.

Your heave contains blood or what looks like coffee grounds.

You have trouble breathing.

Is it heartburn or a heart attack?

Heartburn does n't affect your heart, but it can feel a lot like the casket pain that happens during a heart attack. Call 911 if you have any of these symptoms along with casket pain, indeed if you're not sure that you 're having a heart attack

Dizziness

Nausea and puking

Pain that travels to your neck and shoulder, jaw, or back

Briefness of breath

Sweating

Untoward Heartburn Relief

Type of drug how they work how presto they start working how long the goods last Side goods

Antacids

They neutralize stomach acid. Within seconds Up to 3 hours Some beget constipation and diarrhea.

They lower the quantum of acid your stomach makes. In about 30 twinkles Up to 12 hours

They may beget constipation, diarrhea, headache, nausea, or puking.

Proton- Pump Impediments (PPIs)

They lower the quantum of acid your stomach makes. Up to 4 days Up to 24 hours

They may beget diarrhea, headache, stomach pain, nausea, or puking.

Constipation

How do I know if I 'm constipated?

What's considered a normal number of bowel movements varies from person toperson. However, you're presumably constipated, If you're straining when going to the restroom. You may also have hard droppings or a feeling that your bowel movement is n't complete.

Occasional constipation is common, but if you have lower than three bowel movements in a week, see your croaker

What causes it?

There are numerous causes of constipation, and occasionally you have further than one

Not drinking enough water

Eating a diet low in fiber

Traveling or changing your routine

Getting too little exercise

Taking certain drugs, similar as antidepressants, antihistamines, iron, and some pain specifics (particularly narcotic pain specifics)

Medical conditions including cancer, diabetes, IBS, and hypothyroidism

gestation

Blockages in the large intestine

Problems with the jitters or muscles around the large intestine or rectum

Taking too numerous laxatives

How can I help and treat constipation without drug?

Drink plenitude of water (60- 80 ounces per day). A redundant two to four spectacles a day may help.

Eat prunes or bran cereal to get 20- 35 grams of fiber per day. Eat further vegetables and fruit.

 Drink warm water or herbal tea in the morning.

Exercise frequently.

What OTC specifics can I take for constipation?

When life changes do n't break your problems, several over-the-counter specifics can help. Talk to your druggist or croaker about which drug is right for you. Be sure to read markers precisely before taking these drugs. Using some untoward treatments for constipation for further than 2 weeks can make your symptoms worse and may be a sign of commodity more serious.

Bulk- forming laxatives. You take these fiber supplements with water to bulk up your coprolite, which can spark your intestine to push it out. Some common bulk laxatives are methylcellulose, polycarbophil, psyllium, and wheat dextrin.

Lubricants, like mineral oil painting. They cover the face of the intestine and block water from being absorbed from the coprolite, which helps it pass more fluently.

Bibulous agents. These help keep further water in the intestine, which can expand the intestine and stimulate a bowel movement. Bibulous agents aren't for some aged grown-ups and people with heart or order failure. Talk to your croaker before taking this type of drug.

Coprolite mufflers. By adding fluid to droppings, mufflers help you avoid straining and make them easier to pass instigations. These laxatives make the bowel contract, which helps move the coprolite.

Suppositories or enemas. Some laxatives come in a form that can be fitted into the rectum. These are helpful when you have to avoid straining, similar as after surgery or parturition.

Hemorrhoids

What are hemorrhoids?
Hemorrhoids are blown blood vessels in the rectum and the anus, and they can be uncomfortable. They can be either inside the rectum (internal) or under the skin around the anus(external). Internal hemorrhoids generally do n't beget discomfort, though straining to have a bowel movement may beget them to bleed or lead to spasms in the muscles of the rectum, which can be painful. External hemorrhoids itch and may bleed.
What are the symptoms of hemorrhoids?
Bleeding during a bowel movement. You might also notice blood on the restroom paper after you wipe.
Itching around the anus
lump or pain around the anus
Painful or sensitive lumps around the anus
If you suppose you have hemorrhoids. Bleeding can also be a symptom of commodity more serious.

What causes hemorrhoids?

Constipation or straining during bowel movements causes utmost hemorrhoids. You may also have hemorrhoids if you do not get enough fiber in your diet.
Being pregnant or fat can beget hemorrhoids because of the redundant pressure on your rectum. Hormonal changes that be during gestation can also weaken the muscles of the rectum and anus.

You're also more likely to get them if you sit for long ages of time. And they are more common as you get aged. Other causes include having diabetes, a once rectal surgery, and colon cancer.

When should I call my croaker?

If you suppose you have hemorrhoids. They can recommend treatment and make sure your symptoms aren't caused by another condition.

You should also see your croaker

If your hemorrhoids have n't gotten better with treatment. You may need to see a croaker

Who specializes in hemorrhoids?

How can I treat hemorrhoids without drug?

Add fiber to your diet to help relieve constipation and make your droppings softer. This will make it easier to have bowel movements and reduce the pressure on hemorrhoids.

Try a coprolite quieter.

Exercise to help relieve constipation.

Do n't strain during bowel movements.

Soak in a plain, warm bath or sit bath (a many elevation of water that covers your private corridor and bottom) to help relieve the pain

Keep the area clean and dry.

Use wettish wipes rather of dry restroom paper so you do n't irritate the area any farther.

Apply an ice pack or cold wave compress to help with swelling.

Avoid racy foods to help itching.

Which OTC specifics treat hemorrhoids?

Specifics include creams, suppositories, pads, and ointments. Utmost products contain witch hazel or hydrocortisone, which can help stop the itching and swelling and may ease pain. Utmost over-the-counter specifics shouldn't be used for further than a week. Talk to your croaker or druggist about which is the stylish option for you.

Diarrhea

What's diarrhea?
Diarrhea is loose, watery coprolite that sends you to the restroom more frequently than usual. When you have diarrhea, you may have stomach pain and cramps or bloating.
What causes it?
Numerous effects beget diarrhea, including contagions, bacteria, spongers, specifics, and medical conditions that affect the stomach, bowel, or colon. What you eat can also be a malefactor. Still, mild diarrhea, there's presumably no reason for concern, If you have occasional. But if it lasts for further than 2 days and has n't bettered, you should call your doctor. However, call your pediatrician, if your child or child has diarrhea.
If you have diarrhea along with any of these symptoms;

      v Severe belly or rectal pain
      v Bloody or black droppings
      v Fever above 102 F

Dehumidification. Signs of dehumidification include feeling veritably thirsty, having a dry mouth or skin, having little or no urine, having dark unheroic urine, and feeling weak.
How can I treat my diarrhea?
Drink plenitude of fluids (water, sports drinks, fruit juice) to keep from getting dehydrated. Avoid alcohol, caffeine, and dairy. However, you can eat straight, mellow, if you are n't revolted.

As long as you do n't have other symptoms that worry you, you may also try some untoward treatments
Loperamide (Imodium)This comes in liquid and capsules. It works by decelerating movement in your bowel and colon so

you can absorb further water, making the coprolite less watery. Talk to your croaker about taking this drug. Don't give it to children under 2.

Bismuth subsalicylate (Pepto- Bismol, Pink Bismuth) This drug reduces mild diarrhea and comes in liquids, capsules, and chewable tablets. You should n't take it if you 're antipathetic to aspirin or have a fever. Do n't give it to children under 2. still, do n't take this drug before talking to your croaker if you 're taking a blood thinner.

Probiotics The same supplements that can help with bloating from gas may also help relieve some types of diarrhea by adding "good " bacteria to your digestive system. Sources include;

v Apples
v Citrus fruits
v Lentils
v Nuts
v Oatmeal
v Psyllium

Undoable fiber does n't dissolve in water. Suppose of it as a broom it helps keep food and waste moving through your body. Because undoable fiber attracts water in your gut, it makes droppings softer and easier to pass. Eating a diet rich in undoable fiber can help with constipation.
Sources include;

v Carrots
v Cauliflower
v Legumes
v Potatoes
v Whole grains

Women should get about 25 grams of fiber per day. Men should get 38 grams.
Drinking water
Water is essential to good health and normal bowel function. Water also helps keep droppings soft but solid and well-formed. Avoid drinking potables similar as coffee or soda pop if you suppose they spark your digestive problems.

Probiotics

Your digestive tract is full of different kinds of bacteria. You may suppose that's a bad thing, but utmost of the bacteria in your gut are healthy. They break down poisons, help your body make some vitamins, and play a part in keeping you healthy. But when you have too important of some kinds of bacteria, you may get an illness or have unwelcome symptoms.

Probiotics are like the healthy bacteria in your body. Eating foods that contain them, or taking probiotic supplements, can help keep a balance of good and bad bacteria in your body.
Experts are n't sure exactly how they work, but probiotics may help

- v Relieve bloating from gas
- v Keep you regular
- v Relieve some types of diarrhea
- v Boost your impunity
- v Fight infections
- v help dangerous bacteria from growing in your stomach
- v Destroy the bacteria that make you sick
- v Make B vitamins your body needs

Which foods contain probiotics?
Buttermilk
Fermented and unfermented milk
Kefir
Kimchi
Miso
Sauerkraut
Some pickles
Some soft crapola

Soy drinks
Tempeh
Yogurt with live, active societies
Should I take a probiotic supplement?
People with certain conditions should n't take them, and some probiotics may affect how well your other specifics work or druggist about whether probiotic supplements are right for you.
As soon as food enters the body through the mouth, the process of digestion begins.
The body gradationally moves it through the digestive system, which breaks the food down into lower, more useable corridor.
Colorful foods can help at different stages of this process. For illustration, some aid digestion in the stomach, while others support the bowel.
Fiber is essential to digestive health in general. However, it's stylish to increase fiber input sluggishly, starting with answerable fiber similar as from oatmeal, If a person isn't used to eating fiber frequently.

 Add around one serving of fiber to the diet every 4 – 5 days.
Adding fiber input too snappily can be bad for digestion.
Drinking plenitude of water is also important, as it combines with fiber and adds bulk to coprolite.
Specific foods that are good for digestion include;
Foods containing gusto

Gusto is a factory that can reduce bloating and other digestive problems.
Dried gusto greasepaint is an excellent spice for seasoning refections, and a person can also use slices of gusto root to make tea.

Choose a quality gusto root greasepaint for seasoning refections. For tea, choose fresh gusto root for the stylish results.

Unsaturated fats

This type of fat helps the body absorb vitamins. It also combines with fiber to help encourage bowel movements.
Factory canvases similar as olive oil painting are a good source of unsaturated fats.

Always consume fats in temperance. For an adult following a 2,000- calorie- per- day diet, for illustration, fat input shouldn't exceed 77 grams daily.

Vegetables with skin

Vegetables are rich in fiber, which is an important nutrient for digestion. Fiber stimulates the intestine to move coprolite out of the body.
The skins of vegetables are frequently rich in fiber, and it's stylish to consume them whole. Some vegetables with skin rich in fiber include potatoes, sap, and legumes.

Fruits

Numerous fruits are also rich in fiber. They also contain vitamins and minerals that are good for digestion, similar as vitamin C and potassium.
For illustration, apples, oranges, and bananas are nutritional fruits that could help with digestion.

Whole- grain foods

Whole- grain foods also have a high fiber content that aids digestion. The body breaks down whole grains sluggishly, which helps control blood sugar situations.
Numerous whole grain foods are available, including brown rice and quinoa.

Yogurt

Numerous yogurt products contain probiotics. These are live bacteria and provocations that may have benefits for the digestive system.

Kefir

Kefir is a fermented milk drink that's filling and contains probiotics. As mentioned over, these may promote better digestion and gut health.
What to avoid
Eating too presto may hinder digestion.
Although utmost foods are fine to consume in temperance, some aren't as helpful for digestion.
Some foods and drinks increase the threat of bloating, heartburn, and diarrhea. Exemplifications of these trusted Source include;

v Artificial sweeteners, similar as sugar alcohols
v Carbonated potables or sugar candied drinks
v Refined carbohydrates, similar as white chuck

Some habits can also hinder digestion. These include eating too presto and lying down incontinently after eating.
The body can also take longer to digest large refections, which may be problematic for some people. To enhance digestion, it's stylish to eat several small refections rather of one large bone.
Utmost foods that enhance digestion are rich in nutrients similar as fiber. Exemplifications of fiber-rich foods include vegetables and whole grains.
Some people prone to digestive issues may profit from eating lower refections, as well as consuming a healthy quantum of fiber and avoiding any detector foods.

Conclusions

The second element that is significantly linked to getting older after age is health loss. The stereotypical idea is that everyone higher than a certain age is ill and relies on others for their care. That illustration serves as an example in the discussion of the growing expense of healthcare.